Copyright © 2024 by De Janét Bailey. All rights reserved.

No part of this book may be reproduced, distributed, or transmitted in any form or by any means, including photocopying, recording, or other electronic or mechanical methods, without the prior written permission of the publisher, except in the case of brief quotations embodied in critical reviews and certain other noncommercial uses permitted by copyright law. For permission requests, write to the publisher, addressed "Attention: Permissions Coordinator," at the email address below.

De Janét Bailey

ratewithcare@gmail.com

Enhancing Clinical Instruction: Post-Conference Activities for Effective Teaching

De Janét Bailey, MSN, RN, FNP-C

"I am because we are"-Ubuntu

Table of Contents

Introduction	4
Activity 1 Reflection	5
Activity 2 ISBAR Communication Tool	8
Activity 3 Practice NCLEX Style Questions	10
Activity 4 Supply Room Quest	12
Activity 5 Hand-off Report	14
Activity 6 Role-play	16
Activity 7 Assignment Management	18
Activity 8 Interpretation of EKG Strips	24
Activity 9 Interprofessional Collaboration	26
Activity 10 Hot Topics	27
Activity 11 Case Studies	29
Unit Assignment Sheets	30
Acknowledgement	36

Enhancing Clinical Instruction: Post-Conference Activities for Effective Teaching

My name is De Janét Bailey, MSN, RN, FNP-C, and I have served as a clinical nursing instructor for students pursuing a Bachelor of Science in Nursing degree. Through my experience, I have recognized the critical importance of aligning clinical objectives with innovative post-conference activities to sustain student engagement. It is essential for clinical nursing instructors to foster successful student outcomes by encouraging continuous learning and providing constructive feedback.

This book aims to function as a valuable reference guide for post-conference clinical activities. During the post-conference phase, the clinical instructor's role is to facilitate a learning environment that encourages reflection, active participation in discussions, critical thinking development, and peer collaboration. Serving as a clinical instructor presents a vital opportunity to shape the development of the next generation of nurses. When implementing any post-conference activity, it is important to continuously assess each student's learning needs and tailor activities to their respective academic levels. By doing so, instructors can ensure that the activities are both challenging and achievable, thereby maximizing the educational benefits for all students involved.

Establishing a conducive learning atmosphere enhances students' knowledge and confidence, enabling them to effectively apply theoretical concepts in practice and prepare for their future roles as professional nurses. By offering various engaging and reflective activities, clinical nursing instructors can support their students' growth, enhance their clinical skills, and prepare them for successful careers within the nursing field. The objective of this book is to offer clinical nursing instructors a comprehensive outline of various post-conference activities designed to enhance student engagement and learning within the clinical environment.

Activity One: Reflection

Purpose: Enable students to debrief and articulate their clinical experiences to pinpoint gaps in knowledge and skills.

Benefits: Enhance clinical judgment, receive valuable support and feedback from both instructors and peers, and reflect on clinical events.

Reflective activities such as journaling, clinical debriefing, and simulation debriefing are crucial for professional growth. Journaling encourages students to document their clinical experiences, thoughts, and emotions. By writing regularly, students can develop self-awareness and identify patterns in their learning and practice. Instructors can review the journals and provide personalized feedback, helping students set goals and track their progress over time. This activity provides instructors with an opportunity to identify strengths and areas of improvement for each student.

Clinical and simulation debriefing sessions help students internalize lessons learned and apply them in future clinical situations. The clinical instructor will facilitate a group discussion by posing open-ended questions that provide constructive feedback and encourage individual and collective reflection to enhance learning outcomes. Each student will have an opportunity to discuss their performance, reflect on what went well, and identify areas of improvement. Reflecting on patient assignments and interactions with patients, families, and staff helps students navigate through daily dilemmas experienced by healthcare professionals. Additionally, this activity enables the clinical instructor to identify knowledge gaps and offer constructive feedback to help students navigate clinical scenarios. The next page provides a list of potential reflection questions to consider during the post-conference discussion. By discussing these questions, students can deepen their understanding, support each other's learning, and develop a reflective practice that is essential for their growth as competent and compassionate healthcare professionals.

Reflection Questions:

1. What were your initial thoughts or feelings after reviewing your clinical assignment?
2. What aspects of your clinical day went well?
3. What was a significant challenge you faced during your clinical experience today, and how did you address it?
4. What are your expectations for your role as a student nurse?
5. How would you define the role of a nurse?
6. In what ways did your plan evolve throughout the clinical day?
7. What challenges did the nursing staff face during your shift?
8. How did the situation impact your feelings?
9. What are my strengths and weaknesses?
10. What improvements could have been made during that event?
11. How would you respond if faced with a similar situation in the future?
12. What skills or knowledge did you gain from this experience?
13. How did you incorporate patient-centered care in your interactions, and what was the outcome?
14. Can you share an instance where teamwork played a crucial role in patient care? What did you learn from this experience?
15. Describe a situation where effective communication made a difference in patient care or team collaboration.
16. Reflect on a moment when you felt particularly empathetic towards a patient or their family. How did this impact your approach to care?

17. What strategies did you use to manage stress or anxiety during your shift? How effective were they?

18. Discuss the clinical skills or procedures you performed today. What went well, and what could be improved?

19. How did you ensure patient safety during your clinical activities?

20. Share a lesson learned from observing or interacting with a healthcare professional today. How will you apply this lesson in your future practice?

21. Reflect on the feedback you received from your clinical instructor or peers. How will you use this feedback to enhance your clinical skills and knowledge?

Activity Two: ISBAR Communication Tool

Purpose: Encourage use of the Introduction/Identify, Situation, Background, Assessment, and Recommendation (ISBAR) communication tool in clinical settings to help students organize their thoughts and pinpoint essential patient information for effective communication.

Benefits: Enhances critical thinking, structures communication, fosters teamwork, and boosts student confidence.

To help students become proficient with the ISBAR communication tool, clinical instructors should ensure that students practice it daily within the clinical environment. Since communication is a vital aspect of the nursing profession, it is essential for students to learn how to effectively utilize the ISBAR framework. The clinical and post-conference setting provides ideal opportunities for students to implement this tool.

There are several ways instructors can incorporate the use of ISBAR. First, instructors can set the expectation for students to present their daily patient cases to the group using the ISBAR format. Each day students will be encouraged to report on their patient assignments using the ISBAR communication tool. After each presentation, both students and the instructor will provide constructive feedback on any information that could have been beneficial or omitted. Questions will be posed to ensure a comprehensive understanding of the patient's situation.

Another effective way to promote the use of the ISBAR tool is through scenario-based activities, such as emergency situations, hand-off reports, communication with healthcare providers, and interactions with family members. These scenarios allow students to identify key information and discuss the rationale for including or omitting details based on the context. Students will also learn how the ISBAR framework helps communicate concise information. For instance, an instructor could create a scenario requiring a student to contact the attending physician due to a sudden change in the patient's condition. The student would then deliver information using the ISBAR format and receive telephone orders from the provider. The instructor could add a creative twist by withholding certain information when issuing orders to test the student's ability to identify discrepancies and request necessary information.

ISBAR:

Introduction/Identify: Introduce yourself, identify the patient, and specify the location.

Situation: Describe what is happening with the patient and clearly outline the problem.

Background: Provide relevant clinical background or context, including brief and pertinent information related to the situation.

Assessment: State your professional conclusion based on the situation and background, articulating what you believe the problem to be.

Recommendation: Specify what action you are requesting or recommending.

Activity Three: NCLEX Practice Questions

Purpose: Increase exposure to various NCLEX-style questions to prepare students for the exam.

Benefits: Early preparation for the NCLEX exam, development of clinical reasoning skills, application of knowledge, identification of students' understanding of content, and identification of strengths and weaknesses.

For this activity, select NCLEX practice questions that are related to topics students have previously or are currently discussing within the didactic portion of the course. Remember, clinical is not the time to introduce students to a new topic, so align all post-conference activities with the course schedule provided in the syllabus. During my experience, most students were open about discussing the outcomes of a recent exam or assignment. Their transparency made it more feasible to formulate a consensus on NCLEX study topics to focus on during the post-conference session. Practicing NCLEX-style questions during post-conference is a great opportunity to facilitate discussion and expand on students' current level of knowledge.

The clinical instructor may get creative by practicing NCLEX-style questions during post-conference. I utilized an NCLEX-style Prep App to assist students with practice questions and discussion of rationales; there are various NCLEX-style preparation books and apps on the market. For this activity, students will answer each question as a group and are allotted time to discuss answers with one another. The main goal of this activity is to make it enjoyable for students; they should not feel as if they are taking a didactic exam or quiz. Emphasize that students may use additional resources to assist in answering the questions, but also challenge each student appropriately. As the clinical instructor, you will eventually gain insight into each student's strengths and weaknesses. Additionally, the clinical instructor can invite each student to choose 3-5 NCLEX-style questions they wish to practice during post-conference. The instructor could make this activity more advanced by encouraging students to create NCLEX-style questions, which fosters autonomy, particularly among senior-level students.

Activity Four: Supply Room Quest

Purpose: Enable students to become acquainted with the items available in the supply room.

Benefits: Improve patient safety, promote proper use of supplies, and promote teamwork and communication.

This activity is highly advantageous for nursing students at an introductory level. Familiarization with items in the supply room is crucial for several reasons. Firstly, it enhances students' confidence and efficiency when locating and using these items in real-life scenarios. Secondly, understanding each item's purpose and proper use ensures patient safety and improves the quality of care provided. Additionally, this activity fosters a sense of responsibility and accountability among students as they learn to take care of frequently used equipment and supplies. It also aids in inventory management, allowing students to identify when supplies are running low, need replenishing, or have expired. By engaging in this hands-on learning experience, students develop practical skills essential in a clinical setting, preparing them for their future roles as healthcare professionals.

Activity Instructions:

1. Begin with a brief introduction to the supply room, explaining its importance and the types of items stored there.
2. Divide the students into small groups and assign each group a section of the supply room to explore.
3. Provide each group with a list of supplies and labels or tags.
4. Instruct the students to locate each item on their list, attach the appropriate label or tag, and note the item's purpose and proper use.
5. After all items have been identified and labeled, reconvene as a class to discuss the findings.

6. Please encourage students to share any insights or questions about specific supplies.
7. Conclude with a reflection on how this exercise will aid them in their future clinical practice.

Activity Five: Hand-off Report

Purpose: Enhance students' ability to communicate clearly and effectively about patient status.

Benefits: Strengthen communication skills, professionalism, clinical judgment, and promote patient safety.

Familiarity with hand-off reports is essential in the healthcare field. This activity benefits students at all levels and allows the instructor to evaluate their growth. Each student will engage in delivering, receiving, and critiquing hand-off reports. They will identify key components of each report and discuss factors that may influence reporting, such as environmental impacts.

This activity incorporates peer feedback sessions, which will be integral as they provide diverse perspectives and foster a collaborative learning environment. There are multiple practical formats to organize this activity. One option is for the instructor to utilize a round-robin style for hand-off reports, allowing students to convene and present their patients. Another option is for the instructor to facilitate one-on-one practice sessions before regrouping for collective reflection. Students will be encouraged to reflect on their hand-off report by identifying what went well and areas for improvement. Students will have the chance to ask questions and demonstrate how to give a hand-off report, including:

- What information is relevant?
- How do we involve the patient in the report?
- What bedside checks should be performed?
- What safety checks should be implemented?

Students should observe the nurses deliver hand-off reports, which will enable students to recognize and appreciate the essential information that should be communicated.

By engaging in this structured practice, students will better understand the nuances of patient hand-offs, leading to improved patient care. Active participation will teach them to communicate succinctly and confidently, ensuring essential information is accurately conveyed.

Simulated patient scenarios can be incorporated to enhance realism and provide context. These simulations can range from common clinical situations to more complex cases, allowing students to practice under varying degrees of pressure and urgency. Role-playing as different healthcare team members will also help students appreciate the importance of each role and how interdisciplinary collaboration enhances patient outcomes. This comprehensive approach ensures that students not only master the technical aspects of hand-off reporting but also develop the soft skills necessary for effective communication.

Activity Six: Role-play

Purpose: Ensure students are equipped with realistic scenarios that they may encounter in their professional practice.

Benefits: Enhances communication skills, improves problem-solving abilities, promotes collaboration, builds empathy, and allows students to practice clinical skills in a safe environment. Promotes comfort and confidence by managing the unpredictability of real patient interactions.

Role-playing exercises offer another dynamic approach to post-conference activities. Incorporating role-play into the post-conference curriculum prepares students for the technical aspects of their jobs. It equips them with the soft skills necessary to provide compassionate and effective patient care. Students can practice their communication and interpersonal skills in a safe and supportive environment by simulating patient-nurse interactions. This method helps build confidence and prepares students for real-world clinical encounters. Instructors can create various scenarios that reflect common challenges nurses face, allowing students to explore different strategies and solutions. The instructor can organize the role-play scene in an empty hospital room or in a simulation lab at the facility. Assign each student a specific role such as the patient, nurse, or physician to simulate real-life clinical environments. This hands-on approach can help solidify theoretical knowledge through practical application.

Interactive simulation sessions are another method to introduce students to role-play. By simulating real-life situations, students can learn to manage stress and make informed decisions under pressure. Interactive simulation sessions also provide an opportunity to focus on specific clinical skills, such as patient communication, medication administration, or wound care. This allows students to obtain hands-on experience and deepen their understanding of specific skills and topics. Simulation sessions can be supplemented with multimedia resources to cater to diverse learning styles.

In the end, role-play and familiarization activities are indispensable components of nursing education. They bridge the gap between theoretical knowledge and practical application and prepare students to face the complexities of healthcare with confidence and competence.

Activity Instructions:

1. Divide students into groups and assign roles such as physician, nurse, patient, or family member. Assigning students various roles helps them understand different perspectives and responsibilities.

2. Create a realistic scenario that the students might encounter in their professional practice. Ensure it is detailed enough to allow for meaningful engagement.

3. Clearly outline the learning objectives for the role-play session. This ensures students know which skills or knowledge they should focus on.

4. Allow students to act out the scenario, providing them with the opportunity to practice communication, decision-making, and clinical skills in a controlled environment.

5. After the role-play, hold a debriefing session where students can discuss what went well, what challenges they faced, and how they can improve. This reflection is crucial for the improvement of learning outcomes.

Activity Seven: Assignment Management

Purpose: Examine the complexities and processes of creating a staffing assignment that ensures safe and efficient patient care.

Benefits: Encourages the development of critical thinking and decision-making abilities.

Divide students into groups and provide each group with an assignment sheet containing details about staffing, patient numbers, patient acuity, and safety considerations. Use a blank assignment sheet from the current clinical site. I have created a unit assignment sheet to give you a visual reference for this activity. If you would like to create your own scenario, blank unit assignment sheets have been provided beginning on page 30. I highly recommend using the unit assignment sheet from your assigned clinical department. Ensure the staffing mix includes RNs, LPNs, and new graduate RNs, enabling students to explore and discuss various scopes of practice and expertise levels. To enhance engagement, introduce hypothetical scenarios that challenge their critical thinking skills. Facilitate a discussion on the importance of effective communication with the house supervisor and staffing office. Encourage students to present their staffing plans to the class, fostering an environment where peer feedback can be shared constructively. This collaborative approach enhances learning and mirrors real-world healthcare settings where teamwork and communication are paramount.

Hypothetical Scenario Questions:

- How would the assignment sheet be adjusted if an RN called off their shift?
- What changes would occur if a CNA arrived 1-2 hours late for their shift?
- How would the assignment differ if a nurse were mentoring a new graduate during the shift?
- How would you distribute the patient load based on the available staff?

- Who should be contacted regarding any of the scenarios above, and why?
- Discuss the roles of the house supervisor versus the staffing office.

After each group presents, engage the class in a reflective discussion. Ask students to consider:

- What were the strengths and weaknesses of each group's plan?
- How did each group prioritize patient safety and care quality?
- Were there any innovative approaches or strategies that stood out?
- How might the plans differ in various clinical settings, such as a busy emergency department versus a long-term care facility?

Additionally, integrate a debriefing session where students can discuss the emotional and ethical aspects of staffing decisions. This can include topics such as:

- The impact of staffing shortages on patient care and staff well-being.
- Ethical dilemmas that may arise when resources are limited.
- Strategies for advocating for better staffing and support within their future workplaces.

By addressing these broader themes, students can develop a more comprehensive understanding of the complexities involved in staffing assignments. They will also be better prepared to manage the multifaceted challenges they will encounter in their nursing careers.

Finally, provide resources such as articles, guidelines, and case studies related to effective staffing and patient care. Encourage students to stay informed and continue learning about the best nurse management and leadership practices. This ongoing education will empower them to make informed, ethical, and practical decisions in their professional practice.

Unit Assignment Sheet

Department	Staff
4B	1 Charge nurse: Alpha 4 RNs: Nurse A, Nurse B, Nurse C, Nurse D (New graduate) 1 LPN: Nurse E 2 CNAs: CNA 1, CNA 2 1 unit clerk: Beta

Room	Nurse	CNA	Acuity Level	Safety Precautions	Notes
100	Nurse A	CNA 1	Q4H vitals, wound care, Altered mental status	Contact/fall risk	
101	Nurse A	CNA 1	Total care		
102	Nurse A	CNA 1	Blood transfusion	Neutropenic precautions	
103	Nurse A		Pending discharge		
104	Nurse B			Suicide precautions	

105	Nurse B		Pending Admission		
106	Nurse B			Airborne	
107	Nurse B				
108	Nurse C			Fall risk, seizure	
109	Nurse C			Droplet	
110	Nurse C		Pending admission		
111	Nurse C		Independent		
112	Nurse D		Independent, Q8H vitals		
113	Nurse D		PCA, chest tube		

114	Nurse D		Q2H turn, total care	Fall risk	
115	Nurse D		Central lines, Blood transfusion, PEG tube	Fall risk	
116	Nurse D		Heparin infusion	Droplet	
117	Nurse E		Total Care	Fall risk	
118	Nurse E		Pending discharge to rehab facility		Discharge scheduled for 1300
119	Nurse E		Pain management		
120	Nurse E		Pending Admission		

This unit assignment sheet serves as an excellent illustration of an assignment sheet designed without considering patient acuity and staff experience levels. Instead, it was developed primarily based on convenience and proximity of rooms. It is crucial to highlight that assignments should extend beyond mere room proximity. Typically, assignments are formulated based on factors such as patient acuity, continuity of care, and nursing workload. The nurse-to-patient ratio is a key consideration. This presents a valuable opportunity to explore national guidelines regarding nurse-to-patient ratios, which can differ depending on the state and type of unit. Additionally, discussing legislation that influences these ratios is particularly relevant for students in leadership courses.

Activity Eight: Interpretation of EKG Strips

Purpose: Provide students with the capability to identify normal and abnormal heart rhythms.

Benefits: Improve confidence with rhythm interpretation and increase knowledge related to medication management for abnormal rhythms.

Activity Instructions:

1. Organize students into groups of 2-3 and provide each group with an EKG strip.
2. Have them collaborate to analyze the strip and identify the rhythm.
3. Pose questions regarding the anticipated treatments for the identified rhythm.
4. Inquire about the underlying causes of the rhythm as well.
5. Measure intervals, including the PR interval, QRS duration, and QT interval.
6. Discuss the heart's function based on the EKG findings.

The instructor may source EKG rhythm strips from patients in the unit (pending unit approval) or utilize strips from textbooks. Encourage students to use available resources, such as textbooks and online databases, to cross-reference their findings and deepen their understanding of EKG interpretations. Facilitate a discussion afterwards where each group presents their findings to the class, highlighting the rationale behind their conclusions and any challenges they encountered during the analysis.

To enhance learning, consider integrating technology by utilizing EKG simulation software or apps that allow students to practice rhythm identification in a dynamic and interactive manner. Incorporate a variety of rhythm strips, including those that display common arrhythmias such as atrial fibrillation, ventricular tachycardia, and heart blocks. This diversity will help students become familiar with a wide range of scenarios they may encounter in clinical practice. Provide feedback and guidance throughout the activity, ensuring that students understand the nuances of rhythm interpretation and are prepared to apply this knowledge in real-world clinical settings. This comprehensive approach will improve their technical skills and build their confidence in identifying abnormal cardiac rhythms and managing cardiac patients.

Activity Nine: Interprofessional Collaboration

Purpose: Guide students to understand the importance of interdisciplinary collaboration and the impact interdisciplinary collaboration has on patient care.

Benefits: Enhance patient outcomes, promote patient-centered care, and increase knowledge of interdisciplinary responsibilities.

Evaluate students' understanding of interprofessional collaboration through reflective essays, group discussions, and practical simulations. If possible, invite guest speakers from different disciplines to allow students to understand their roles and responsibilities. Have students participate in morning/afternoon interdisciplinary meetings to better understand their role as nurses. Use feedback from guest speakers and interdisciplinary meetings to provide constructive insights into students' performance and areas for improvement. Incorporate role-playing scenarios where students can act out different interdisciplinary team roles to better appreciate the diverse perspectives and contributions each member brings to patient care. Foster open communication and active listening exercises to build trust and mutual respect among team members.

By the end of these activities, students should be able to articulate the significance of interprofessional collaboration, demonstrate effective communication skills, and recognize the positive impact of teamwork on patient outcomes. They will leave with a deeper appreciation for the collaborative nature of healthcare and the vital role each discipline plays in delivering holistic patient-centered care.

Activity Ten: Hot Topics

Purpose: Discuss current events, healthcare policies, and their impact on the nursing profession. Raise awareness on available opportunities that influence reform and discover how their voices can resonate as future nursing leaders.

Benefits: Identify reliable sources, promote healthcare advocacy, and improve critical thinking skills.

The instructor will utilize any state board of nursing (preferably their state of practice) public records to help students understand standards of practice and learn from past errors made by nurses. The instructor will direct students to evidence-based websites, nursing organizations, and Quality and Safety Education for Nurses (QSEN) for additional resources and guidelines that can enrich their educational journey. The instructor will encourage students to engage in healthy discussions to develop critical thinking skills and a deeper understanding of the complexities within the healthcare system.

Activity Instructions:

1. Assign students to research a recent healthcare-related news article. Students will present their findings during class and discuss the implications for nursing practice and patient care. This will help them stay informed and understand the broader context of their profession.
2. Have students work in groups to explore specific healthcare policies. They should analyze the policy's impact on nursing practice, patient outcomes, and the healthcare system. This project can culminate in a presentation or a written report.
3. Organize workshops where students can learn about advocacy strategies, including effectively communicating with policymakers, participating in professional organizations, and utilizing social media for advocacy. Invite guest speakers who are

experienced nurse advocates to share their insights and experiences and provide students with an opportunity to ask questions.

4. Facilitate discussions on the ethical considerations and standards of practice outlined by state boards of nursing. Use real-life case studies to illustrate common mistakes and lessons learned, fostering a culture of continuous improvement and ethical practice.

5. Guide students to explore websites and resources provided by nursing organizations such as the American Nurses Association (ANA), the National League for Nursing (NLN), and the Quality and Safety Education for Nurses (QSEN) initiative. Encourage them to utilize these research and professional development resources to stay current with best practices.

By incorporating these activities, students will not only gain knowledge but also develop the skills necessary to become influential leaders in the nursing field, capable of advocating for positive changes in healthcare policies and practices.

Activity Eleven: Case Studies

Purpose: Examine clinical case studies that enable students to apply the nursing process.

Benefits: Enhance clinical reasoning, analytical abilities, teamwork skills, decision-making capabilities, and knowledge of common patient conditions.

Case studies allow students to analyze real-life scenarios, identify potential problems, and propose evidence-based solutions. The instructor will provide feedback and additional resources to address any gaps in knowledge or skills observed during the case study analysis. This iterative process ensures continuous improvement and prepares students for real-world clinical practice. Analysis of case studies not only reinforces theoretical knowledge but also sharpens critical thinking and decision-making skills.

For this activity, choose case studies that correlate to topics students have previously studied or are currently exploring in the didactic portion of the course. As previously emphasized, post-conference is not intended to introduce new subjects but to build on students' current foundation. Instructors can encourage students to work in small groups to foster peer collaboration and learn through open dialogue. Each group will analyze the selected case study by identifying the patient's symptoms, history, and test results to formulate a nursing diagnosis. Encourage students to develop a care plan that includes intervention strategies, expected outcomes, and rationales for each decision made. After dissecting the case study, reconvene as a class for a comprehensive debriefing session. Encourage students to share their findings, discuss different approaches taken by each group, and reflect on the challenges they faced. This collaborative reflection will help students appreciate diverse perspectives and enhance their critical thinking abilities.

Unit Assignment Sheet

Department	Staff
	Charge nurse: RNs: LPN: CNAs: Unit clerk:

Room	Nurse	CNA	Acuity Level	Safety Precautions	Notes

Unit Assignment Sheet

Department	Staff
	Charge nurse: RNs: LPN: CNAs: Unit clerk:

Room	Nurse	CNA	Acuity Level	Safety Precautions	Notes

Unit Assignment Sheet

Department	Staff
	Charge nurse: RNs: LPN: CNAs: Unit clerk:

Room	Nurse	CNA	Acuity Level	Safety Precautions	Notes

Unit Assignment Sheet

Department	Staff
	Charge nurse: RNs: LPN: CNAs: Unit clerk:

Room	Nurse	CNA	Acuity Level	Safety Precautions	Notes

Unit Assignment Sheet

Department	Staff
	Charge nurse: RNs: LPN: CNAs: Unit clerk:

Room	Nurse	CNA	Acuity Level	Safety Precautions	Notes

Unit Assignment Sheet

Department	Staff				
	Charge nurse: RNs: LPN: CNAs: Unit clerk:				
Room	**Nurse**	**CNA**	**Acuity Level**	**Safety Precautions**	**Notes**

Acknowledgement

Thank you for dedicating your time to read Enhancing Clinical Instruction: Post-Conference Activities for Effective Teaching. Your commitment to improving educational practices and investing in your professional development is truly commendable. We hope the insights and strategies shared in this book will enhance your teaching journey and positively impact the learning experiences of your students.

If you find this content valuable or have any feedback, we would love to hear from you. Please feel free to contact the author via email at ratewithcare@gmail.com. Your thoughts and experiences are important to us as we continue to explore and share effective teaching methodologies. Together, let us strive to create a supportive learning environment that cultivates the next generation of highly skilled professional nurses.

www.ingramcontent.com/pod-product-compliance
Lightning Source LLC
Chambersburg PA
CBHW062236220526
45471CB00009B/3498